Midlife In Your Face, Man!

Midlife Questions for Men

David C. Regester, PhD

Copyright © 1998 by David Regester, Ph.D.

All rights reserved. No portion of this book may be reproduced – mechanically, electronically, or by any other means, including photocopying – without the written permission of the publisher. Printed in the United States of America.

Library of Congress Catalog Card Number: 98-92746

Regester, David
Midlife in Your Face, Man!
1998

ISBN 0-9663238-5-8

DocReeg Publications
4330 44th Street SW
Grandville, Michigan 49418.

First Printing
10 9 8 7 6 5 4 3 2 1

Ordering information on the last page.

I suggest that we need to get men to ask the "right" (read: personally meaningful) questions. Men are natural born problem-solvers. Finding answers to tough questions is much of where men get their sense of personal satisfaction and work fulfillment. Such accomplishments build their self-esteem.

If men would tackle the "right" questions, they would be more likely to resolve their midlife problems, and feel so much better about that "downward slope" — their second half of life.

A man's midlife "crisis" then would become more a phase of creating and growing a new sense of self. It would be one of life's great passages, and hopefully a much more healthy, creative one at that.

I've also learned that men don't really ease their midlife struggles through the advise of "how to" books. Unlike sports, there are no "pro's" of midlife to imitate. It is a highly individual, unique odyssey. Simplistic solutions just won't do. It's off to the woods and every man for himself.

Listen carefully to yourself. You already may be asking the very questions this book poses. Then again, maybe you haven't discovered the questions that are "right" for you. If you haven't, rest assured, this book will put them **"In your face"**.

Yes, your midlife crisis may take a little longer than you want. Yes, you might even feel some emotional pain and suffering. You might even find (god forbid) reading something helps!

That's okay — just don't tell anybody.

So...wrestle with these midlife questions. Take them on. Reflect on them in your spare(!) time. Remember, other men's answers may provide some pretty good hints, but they just won't work for you. Your answers will be unique. You are one of a kind.

Finally, if you really want to tackle these questions, I suggest you call one of your closest buddies, grab the ole' fishin' pole, golf bag, or whatever, take along a cup o' jo, and struggle with these together. Nothin' like a buddy to keep you honest!

And your questions are right here — right **in your face, man!**

— David C. Regester, Ph.D.

Aging

"Middle age is when you suddenly find that your parents are old, your kids are grown up, and you haven't changed."

— *Fred Schoenberg*

If midnight on the clock

signifies the end of your life,

what time does it feel like to

you now?

Do you feel like you're "growing" or "growing older"?

As you grow older, would you rather lose your mind before your body, or your body before your mind?

If you could stay a certain age indefinitely, what age would you choose and why?

Have you rejected, denied, or welcomed midlife?

When was your last "right of passage" and how did you recognize it?

What do you think it means

to "age deeply"?

What has been the most difficult change you have had to deal with during midlife?

What would be your greatest personal satisfaction from living until you were 150 years old?

Do you expect to continue growing through your middle years, and in what ways?

How much longer would you like to live, and why?

Are you too old to change in significant ways?

Awareness

I stopped a middle-aged person in the street and asked, "Do you think the mid-life crisis is a consequence of ignorance or apathy?"

His answer: "I don't know and I don't care."

— Fred Schoenberg

Would you like to believe that nothing is really any different than during the first half of your life?

Do you feel you are on a potentially fulfilling quest, or are you feeling somewhat "lost at sea"?

What questions have you found so important that you continue to ask them of yourself?

Do you feel you are
living a more fulfilling life
than most other
people your age?

With respect to

risk–taking activities, have

you lost or gained courage?

If you were a musical

instrument now in your life,

which one would it be,

and why?

What is the one thing you would miss the most if your house burned down (injuring no one)?

Do you feel trapped in your life? If so, how would you escape if you could?

Do you feel like two or more selves that just don't fit together?

Are you surprised or dismayed by some of your values, thoughts, or actions that somehow seem out of character for you?

Do you find you attend

less to what makes you angry,

and are valuing other

feelings more?

Are there people you still need to forgive in your life?

Body

"The only two things we do with greater frequency in middle age are urinate and attend funerals."

— Fred Schoenberg

Do you feel your chronological age?

What age do you feel?

What bothers you more: a decline in physical functioning or a decrease in physical attractiveness?

Assuming you are taking care of your body, is it primarily for appearance sake, or for your health?

What accommodations or adaptations have you made to hide the effects of aging?

Does your face look your chronological age?

Do you feel that you are too old to gain from exercise?

What parts of your body are aging faster than others?

How much would you spend

to attain a significantly

younger look?

What part of your body would you change to improve your physical appearance? Your physical functioning? Is it possible?

How are you dealing with having to exercise more each year to attain the same, or even less, benefit?

Have you found physical activities (e.g. sports) that will last into old age?

Is there any part of your body

that you haven't accepted yet?

If so, is it time to do so?

Death

"I'm not afraid to die. I just don't want to be there when it happens."

— Woody Allen

If you only had one year to live, what would you change, and why aren't you changing this now?

How would you like to be remembered after you die?

Would you really like to know the exact date of your death?

If, after you died, you could be reborn, what are your fantasies about the kind of life you would want?

What would have to happen in your life in order for you to die feeling fulfilled?

If you could visit any one place before you die, where would it be, and why?

How would you choose to die, if you could control your death?

What would you say will be your personal gift to the world (family, friends, children, etc.) after you have died?

Do you find yourself looking

at obituaries more often?

What conditions would justify your choosing euthanasia or assisted suicide?

If you feel life is too short,

how many more years would

you like to live?

If you were to die today, what unfinished business would you regret not having finished? What do you intend to do about this?

Future

The future isn't what it used to be.

—Anonymous

If you could live out your

dream, what would

you be doing?

Do you believe that most of your meaningful personal growth is behind you?

Are you fulfilled enough

in the present that

you don't depend too much

on the future?

If you took a magic pill that could give you a fully developed skill, talent, or ability, what would you want it to be?

Do you sometimes feel that you never will achieve anything of significance in your life? Have you made peace with this?

If you had no concern whatsoever about other peoples' feelings, what would you do differently?

If a genie in a bottle had the power to answer one question about your future, what would you most want to know?

Is there anything you would still like to do before you die, if you had the courage (time, money, ability, etc.)?

Are you running out of "firsts" (first date, first car, first house, etc.)?

Are you running out of "lasts" (e.g. last marathon run, last roller coaster ride, etc.)?

Health

"To eat is human, to digest divine."

—Charles Copeland

Have your bodily aches and pains and other symptoms yet grabbed your attention?

How do you feel when friends' conversations turn to their latest body symptoms, problems, surgeries, and so forth?

Will you need a medical crisis to motivate you to make the changes you have only thought about thus far?

Are you eating for nourishment, or to fill up a deep sense of emptiness?

Do you find you are doing more to fight against the gradual physical changes of aging, or are you learning to accept them?

Have you fallen prey to any of those pills that promise to restore your youthful vitality?

Has the fine print in health insurance policies become more important to understand these days?

Do you find yourself buying all sorts of nutritional, herbal, or vitamin supplements?

Do you find yourself more willing to try various cosmetic aides to hide your aging, or are you accepting your changes with grace and dignity?

Are you a sucker for the latest weight loss program?

Lifestyle

"I am a deeply superficial person."

— Andy Warhol

Is there a significant lifestyle change you would like to make?

Does your lifestyle allow you to pause and enjoy it?

Do you have a

fulfilling hobby?

Does simplifying your life seem more attractive than previously?

Is keeping up with the Joneses

still a major concern?

Is your life still exciting, or doesn't that really matter as much anymore?

Are the lifestyle changes other middle–aged friends are making becoming more, or less, significant to you?

Do you believe that most of your meaningful life is behind you?

Is your image of success harder to maintain, while more difficult to justify to yourself?

If you got a whole lot of
money, would you actually
become more generous
with it?

Marriage

"Marriage: A master, a mistress and two slaves, making in all, two."

— Ambrose Bierce

What would help your relationship more: having more time with your wife or more time away?

If you were legally required to renew your marriage license every five years, knowing your spouse as you do, would you renew now?

Is the number of common interests and activities you share with your wife decreasing as you grow older?

If there is one thing you could do to improve your relationship with your wife, what would you do?

If there is one thing you would like your wife to do to improve your relationship, what would it be?

Over the next ten years, do you feel your marriage will improve, deteriorate, or remain the same?

Has your sense of loving your spouse deepened over the years, or has it become comfortably stable, without much deepening?

Do you believe your wife has any significant aspects of her life which would shock you now if they were revealed?

Would you have an affair if you absolutely could be guaranteed it would never be known by your wife?

Overall, are you able to express your most authentic feelings about your marriage to your wife, or are you still withholding?

What topics still would result in major disagreement with your spouse if you really talked honestly with each other?

What kinds of things are there that your spouse might want to do, or have, that you really would be against?

Do you have any significant secrets that you don't want your wife to know?

If you won $1,000,000 in the lottery, do you believe the money would significantly affect your relationship in any way?

Memories

If I had my life to live over,

I'd live over a delicatessen.

— Anonymous

From what experience have you grown most in your life?

Do your memories help you feel better or worse about your midlife years?

What was the happiest

moment of your life?

Will your memories of your midlife years be mostly positive or mostly negative?

Do you find you are living more through the memories of your past or through your experience of the present?

What was the most difficult

period/event in your life?

How did you know your parents hit midlife?

About what period of your life

are you most nostalgic?

Have you explored your memories of youth for hints of what's missing, threads you may have lost, passions you may have suppressed?

Do you have any recurring memory and is its repeating nature telling you anything important for your life?

Mentors

People who think they know everything are very irritating to those of us who do.

— *Anonymous*

Do you have a personal relationship with anyone you would consider a person of genuine wisdom?

Do you remember who was your first mentor and why he was so important to you then?

Who do you consider your mentor for your life right now? Why?

Does it concern you that you don't have a close relationship with a mentor now?

Are you having sufficient contact with your mentor, and if not, why not?

Who are your heroes in your life now?

Has your mentor ever let you down or disappointed you in some way?

Which book or quote do you find most significant to guide you in life right now?

Do you admire your mentor more for what he has said, or for how he has lived his life?

Do you have a vague sense that you are now training others, in effect, to take over the job you had when you were younger?

Who would you choose to be your best guide through your midlife years?

Do you have a sense that you should now be a mentor to younger men?

Money

"I'm living so far beyond my income that we may almost be said to be living apart."

— *e. e. cummings*

Are you willing to work harder than you are now just to make more money?

Have you discovered that materialistic measures of success (e.g. income) just do not have the same level of fulfillment as before?

Has your pursuit of money left you with a sense that you have neglected large undeveloped parts of yourself?

Are there any words of wisdom, taken from your experience, that you could offer others about the use of money?

Are you earning what

you are worth?

Which would you work harder for: more money or more time off?

Have you made any financial decisions about which you would feel ashamed if they became public knowledge?

Do you find you are giving more or less money or time than you used to give to charities and religious groups?

Have you found that "balance point" between giving to yourself and giving to others?

If you won a large sum of money, would you feel the need to give some of it away, even if no one knew you did?

Parenting

The best revenge is to live long enough to be a problem to your children

— Anonymous

Have you completed your work as a father, or is there still work you need to do?

What would you do differently with your children if you could raise them again?

What comments of personal significance have you passed on to your children in recent months?

How would you feel

about your wife becoming

pregnant now?

Now that your children are out of your house, do you feel more or less willing to take risks?

What regrets do you have about the way you fathered your children?

Are you aware of any sustaining negative effects your parents still have on you?

Have you experienced any significantly negative results of your parenting from your children?

Would you care to raise another child now that you are in midlife?

Have you ever experienced your child being a parent to you in a way that significantly influenced you?

Regrets

"Middle age is like getting an invitation to a great party and then discovering the party was yesterday."

— *Fred Schoenberg*

Do you regret more your missed opportunities or your under-developed personal relationships?

If you could relive any life event, but change it to be the way you wish it were, what would this be?

Are you more regretful about your failure from trying something, or your lack of trying something?

Which period of your life would you like to repeat, if you could?

What is the thing you've done

that you most regret?

What is the thing you've not done that you most regret?

Is there any one thing which stands out in your memory as something you now regret doing, saying, etc. with your parents?

Have your adult children (if any) told you of any regrets they had growing up with you?

Do you regret not having maintained closer lifetime friendships with your childhood and young adult friends?

Assuming you have the power, is there any one thing in your personal history you would like to have prevented?

Relationships

"Anyone who says he can see through women is missing a lot."

— Groucho Marx

What do you need in a best friend, and do you have one?

Do you have friends now who you think still will be very important to you in 10 or 20 years?

Do you think your friends like you because you are successful, or because of your more personal attributes?

Have you ever known

a man who qualified to be

your "soulmate"?

A woman?

Is acquiring male friends

harder than it used to be?

How do you deal with

the increasing difficulty

of making new friends

as one ages?

Have you made up for your inevitable loss of friends through making other friends, or through an increase in activities?

Have the reasons you choose your closest friends changed significantly over the years?

Do you give more to your friends, or do you gain more from your friends?

Is there any one person's statements or actions which have significantly influenced your life lately?

Religion

"Forgive, O Lord, my little jokes on thee, and I'll forgive thy great big one on me."

— Robert Frost

Do you believe in a power

greater than yourself?

Describe this power.

Do you believe your life

has a mission?

Have you experienced anything you would call a "spiritual emergency" (crisis of the spirit)?

What would you say

is your ultimate

concern in life?

Are you more, or less, concerned about an afterlife than in previous years?

What would it take to prove to you there is a God?

Do you have more, or fewer, unanswered questions about your religion today than you did 10 years ago?

Do you really believe God is responsible for what happens in life?

Assuming you could have a personal conversation with Jesus (God, Buddha, etc.), what do you feel you should be talking about?

Upon your death, what one question would you like God to ask, the answer to which will determine whether you have "eternal life"?

Have you found a church which will adequately fulfill most of your spiritual needs?

Do you feel more, or less, inclined to discuss your religious beliefs with others than when you were younger?

What would you say

to God to make your case for

your "eternal reward"?

Are you convinced that good will win over evil in the world, or vice versa?

Retirement

At this age we are wise enough to know that wisdom does not come with age.

—Anonymous

Are you wanting to be the first among your friends to retire, or to be the last?

Do you find yourself unable to apply the word "retirement" to yourself, preferring such words as "rejuvenation, sabbatical, or time off"?

What are your fantasies about your retirement?

Is your inability to live out your values now hastening you to retire sooner?

What age do you feel is acceptable for your full time retirement?

Have you ever seriously considered not retiring?

Do you carry mostly negative images of retirement, e.g. men are more likely to die within their first year, etc.?

Are your fantasies of retirement full of positive images (e.g. hobbies, travel, relaxation) or more just an unknown void?

What do you envision your retirement home will be like?

When you retire, will you be happy with solely personal goals, or will you need to contribute something to society?

Sexuality

"I believe in sex and death – two experiences that come once in a lifetime."

— *Woody Allen*

If your desire has diminished due to natural effects of aging, do you feel your sexual desire is as strong as you would like it to be?

If you, or your wife, but only one of you, could increase your sexual desire a significant amount, which one would you prefer?

How many years

of a good sex life do you

realistically feel you have?

Have you concluded that sex will never again be as good as it once was?

Assuming sex provides less fulfillment than previously, have other forms of intimacy with your wife made up for this loss?

Are there sexual behaviors, roles, or actions which you fantasize about but have not yet tried with your spouse (and may never)?

Is your sexual enjoyment focused more on genital pleasure or more full body pleasure?

How much would you spend to improve the quality of your orgasms?

If for some valid and unchangeable reason, your spouse could never have sexual intercourse again, would this drive you to divorce?

If you could really know your wife's authentic feelings toward you as a sexual lover, would you really want to know?

What frequency of sexual encounters is sufficient for you at this stage in your life?

Would deep feelings of love be sufficient reason to marry now, if you knew you really didn't have any sexual feelings toward your partner?

Assuming your wife is no longer interested in sex, if she accepted your decision, would you satisfy your sexual needs outside your marriage?

Do you think your friends think your sex life is better or worse then theirs? Do you really care what they think?

With your male friends, is it harder to talk about your sex life or your income? Is there any subject more difficult to discuss?

Do you have any "unfinished" sexual business?

Time

"Are you mad? We just had the den redone a couple years ago."

"That was 1968, dear."

— *Fred Schoenberg*

Are you at the end of the first half of your life, or the beginning of your second half?

If you never have enough time, what is it you don't have enough time for?

Does the proportion of time you invest in your daily activities generally represent your life values?

If life were a year long, what month are you in?

Do you feel you can "lighten up", or need to "tighten up", on how you spend your time?

Does time seem to

move faster or slower

to you now?

Have you learned that "slower" is often better than "faster"?

Do you try each day to spend some time engaged in pursuits which are truly of value to you?

Which of your daily activities just are not worth the time anymore – if you were really being honest with yourself?

Do you find yourself measuring your daily activities in terms of how much value each one really is to you?

Values

"Living with a conscience is like driving a car with the brakes on."

— *Budd Schulberg*

Are you listening more to the demands of your head, or your heart?

Have the things which are really important to you significantly changed, or have they largely stayed the same?

Are you satisfied that you honor, and actually live by, a solid sense of ethics?

Would you like to spend more time every day improving your sex life, or your spirituality?

What is your most important

value in life today?

Are you puzzled by your diminished interest in areas of your life that formerly held your interest?

Are you more or less likely to fudge on your income taxes than before?

Are you finding more satisfaction in giving or in receiving?

Do you find yourself donating more time toward helping community causes, or toward projects of purely personal gain?

Do you consider yourself more or less ethical as you grow older?

Work

"Hard work never killed anybody, but why take a chance?"

— Charlie McCarthy (Edgar Bergen)

If you didn't need the money, would you continue to work at your present job?

Do you believe that your career success will lead to your greatest sense of satisfaction in life?

Would you rather have great career success, to the detriment of your private life, or a very fulfilled personal life, to the detriment of your career success?

Is your interest in working primarily due to the intrinsic satisfaction you get from your work?

Is your career your calling?

Assuming no monetary concerns, how much time would you be able to take off from work before you would start getting bored?

If the salary were the same, would you like to try another profession, job, or career?

Is it possible that some alternative value, such as altruism, has surpassed your lifelong investment in the intrinsic value of a productive job?

What is your greatest work accomplishment? Is "accomplishing" still as important?

If you could do it all over again, would you choose your same career?

Bibliography: Midlife Books for Men

Allen, Tim *I'm Not Really Here*. New York: Hyperion, 1996.

Barry, Dave. *Dave Barry Turns 40*. New York: Crown, 1990.

Brehany, Kathleen A. *Awakening at Mid-life: Realizing your Potential for Growth and Change*. New York: Riverhead Books, 1996.

Conway, Jim. *Your Marriage Can Survive Mid-Life Crisis*. Nashville: T. Nelson, 1987

Conway, Jim. *Men in Mid-Life Crisis*. Elgin, Ill.: D.C. Cook Publishing Co., 1978

Colarusso, Calvin A. *Fulfillment in Adulthood: Paths to the Pinnacle of Life*. New Your: Plenum Press, 1994

Goldstein, Ross E. *Fortysomething: Claiming the Power and Passion of your Mid-life Years*. Los Angeles: Jeremy P. Tarcher, 1990

Greene, Bob. *The 50-Year Dash: The Feelings, the Foibles, the Fears of Being a Half-a-century Old*. New York: Doubleday, 1997

Hollis, James. *The Middle Passage: From Misery to Meaning in Mid-life*. Toronto, Canada: Inner City Books, 1988

Johnson, Robert. *He*. New York: Harper & Row, 1974

Johnson, Robert. *Transformation*. New York: Harper & Row, 1991

Levinson, Daniel. *Seasons of a Man's Life*. New York: Alfred A. Knopf, 1978.

Maltland, David Johnston. *Against the Grain: Coming Through Mid-Life Crisis*. New York: Pilgrim Press, 1981

Mayer, Nancy. *The Male Mid-Life Crisis: Fresh Starts After 40*. New York: Doubleday & Co., 1978

Monick, Eugene. *Phallos: Sacred Images of the Masculine*. Toronto, Canada: Inner City Books, 1987

Nolan, WIlliam A. *Crisis Time: Love, Marriage, and the Male at Mid-Life*. New York: Dodd, Mead, 1984

O'Connor, Peter. *Understanding the Mid-Life Crisis*. Melbourne, Australia: Sun Books, 1981

Raines, Howell. *Fly Fishing Through the MidLife Crisis*. New York: William Morrow & Co., 1993

Robinson, John C. *Death of a Hero, Birth of the Soul: Answering the Call of Midlife*. Sacramento, California: Tzedakgh Publications, 1995

Sharp, Daryl. *The Survival Papers: Anatomy of a Midlife Crisis*. Toronto, Canada: Inner City Books, 1988

Sharp, Daryl. *Dear Gladys: The Survival Papers, Book 2*. Toronto, Canada: Inner City Books, 1989

Sheehy, Gail. *Passages*. New York: E.P. Dutton & Co., 1974

Sheehy, Gail. *New Passages*. New York: Random House, 1995

Schoenberg, Fred. *Middle-Age Rage and Other Male Indignities*. New York: Simon & Schuster, 1987

Stein, Murray. *In Midlife*. Dallas, Texas: Spring Publications, 1983

Wyly, James. *The Phallic Quest*. Toronto, Canada: Inner City Books, 1989

Order Form

Fax Orders: (616) 534-2394

Online Orders: docreeg@aol.com

Postal Orders: Doc Reeg Publications
Regester & Associates
4430 44th Street SW
Grandville, MI 49418
(616) 534-6988

Please send _____ copies of **Midlife in Your Face, Man!** to:

Name _____

Address _____

CIty _____ State _____ Zip _____

Telephone (_____) _____

Price per copy @ $9.95 each . . . . _____

Michigan Sales Tax @ 6% ($.60 ea.) . . . . _____

Shipping @ $2.00 each . . . . _____

                Total Included . . . . _____

Please make check payable to "Doc Reeg Publications"

Note: Credit cards not accepted.

Thank You!

Order Form

Fax Orders: (616) 534-2394

Online Orders: docreeg@aol.com

Postal Orders: Doc Reeg Publications
Regester & Associates
4430 44th Street SW
Grandville, MI 49418
(616) 534-6988

Please send _____ copies of **Midlife in Your Face, Man!** to:

Name _____

Address _____

CIty _____ State _____ Zip _____

Telephone (_____) _____

Price per copy @ $9.95 each . . . . _____

Michigan Sales Tax @ 6% ($.60 ea.) . . . . _____

Shipping @ $2.00 each . . . . _____

                    Total Included . . . . _____

Please make check payable to "Doc Reeg Publications"

Note: Credit cards not accepted.

Thank You!

Order Form

Fax Orders: (616) 534-2394

Online Orders: docreeg@aol.com

Postal Orders: Doc Reeg Publications
Regester & Associates
4430 44th Street SW
Grandville, MI 49418
(616) 534-6988

Please send _____ copies of **Midlife in Your Face, Man!** to:

Name _____

Address _____

CIty _____ State _____ Zip _____

Telephone (_____) _____

Price per copy @ $9.95 each . . . . _____

Michigan Sales Tax @ 6% ($.60 ea.) . . . . _____

Shipping @ $2.00 each . . . . _____

                Total Included . . . . _____

Please make check payable to "Doc Reeg Publications"

Note: Credit cards not accepted.

Thank You!